Dear Reader,

We all need our own little BLUEPRINTS, or plans, in life. Sometimes making a plan is fun. Sometimes it's hard. Sometimes the plan doesn't work, so we make a new one. And sometimes, the plan is exactly what we need, just when we need it. As you read this Have a Plan Book, we hope you will ask questions, talk about it with family and friends, and create your very own plan. You can do this on your own or together with a grown-up.

Your plan may grow and change each time you read your book, and that's great! As life happens, plans change. But remember, having a little Blueprint is always helpful, in difficult times and in good times. So go ahead: BLUEPRINT IT!

Lovingly,

Your friends at little BLUEPRINT

P.S. Children and adults around the world are making their own little BLUEPRINTS. If you want to see the plans of others, or share yours, just go to

www.littleBLUEPRINT.com

I0110930

HAVE A PLAN Books

To purchase a hardcover or personalized version of any little BLUEPRINT book, with names, optional photo(s), and details, please go to:

www.littleBLUEPRINT.com

The author would like to thank,
for all of their support and expertise:
Dan Siegel, M.D.;
Nina Shapiro, M.D.;
Sara Ryba, RD, CDN, Founder, www.sararybanutrition.com;
Meredith Liss, MA, RD, CDN, NY Presbyterian Hospital; and
my editor, Leslie Budnick.
A special thanks to
Phoebe, age 10, for her blueprint and title page illustrations.

©2013 little BLUEPRINT. All rights reserved. The contents of this book are copyrighted. Unlawful use of this content, without prior permission, is illegal and punishable by law. Library of Congress Control Number: 2014936210 ISBN 978-1-940101-24-8. little BLUEPRINT and Have a Plan Books are trademarks of little BLUEPRINT, LLC. 1158 26th St., #192, Santa Monica, CA 90403. Printed in the United States.

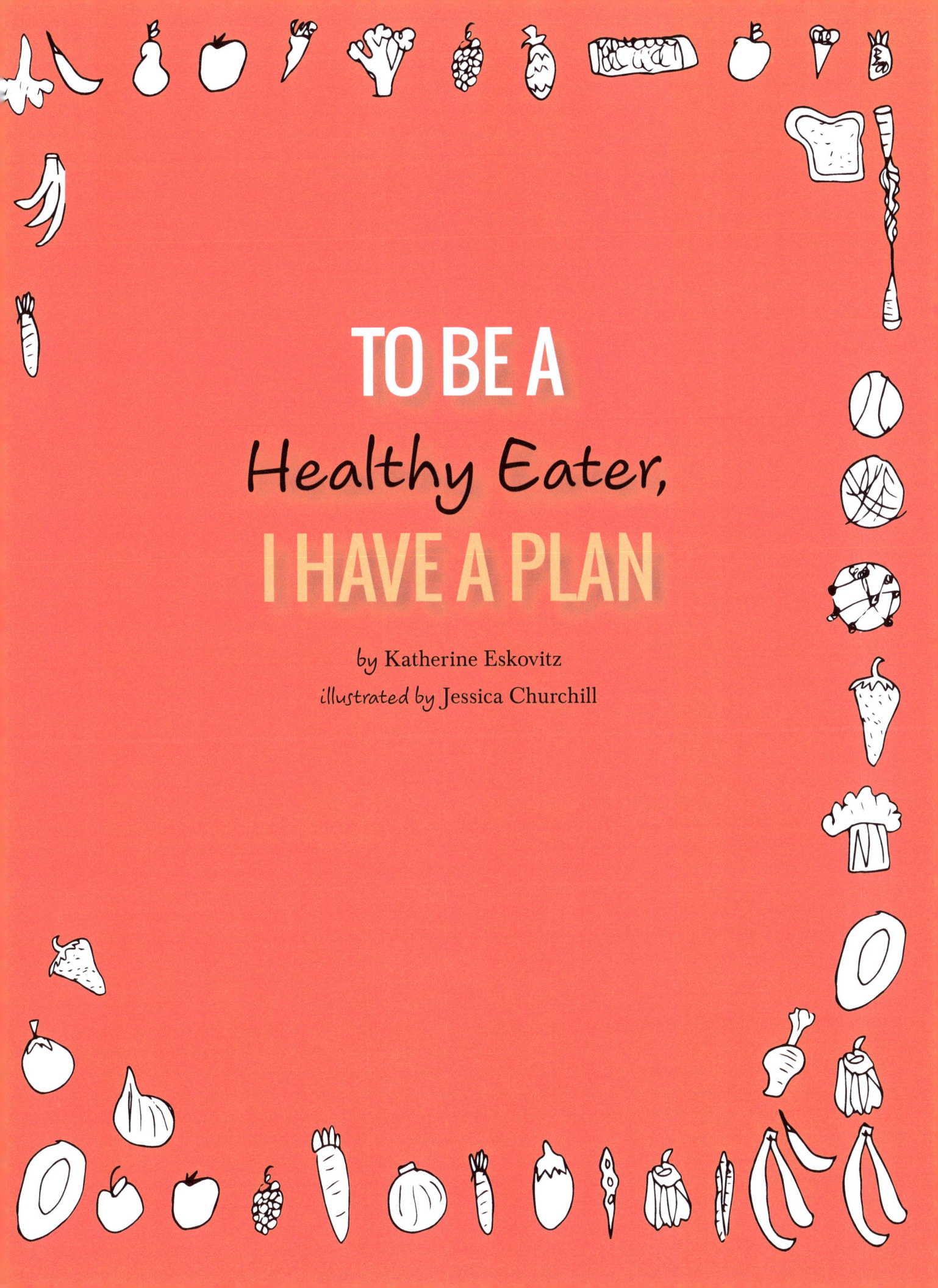

TO BE A
Healthy Eater,
I HAVE A PLAN

by Katherine Eskovitz

illustrated by Jessica Churchill

There is some FOOD that
I really like to eat . . .

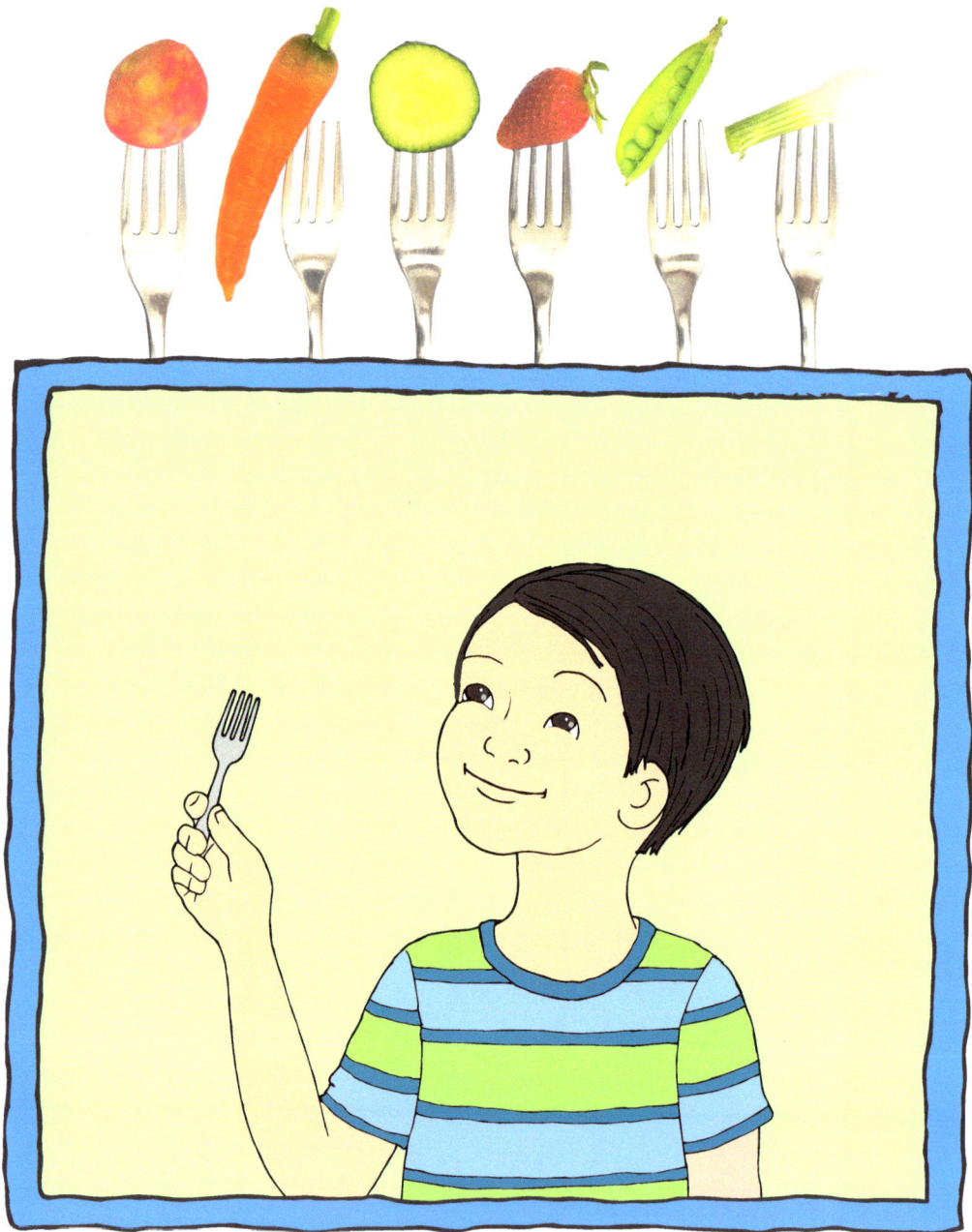

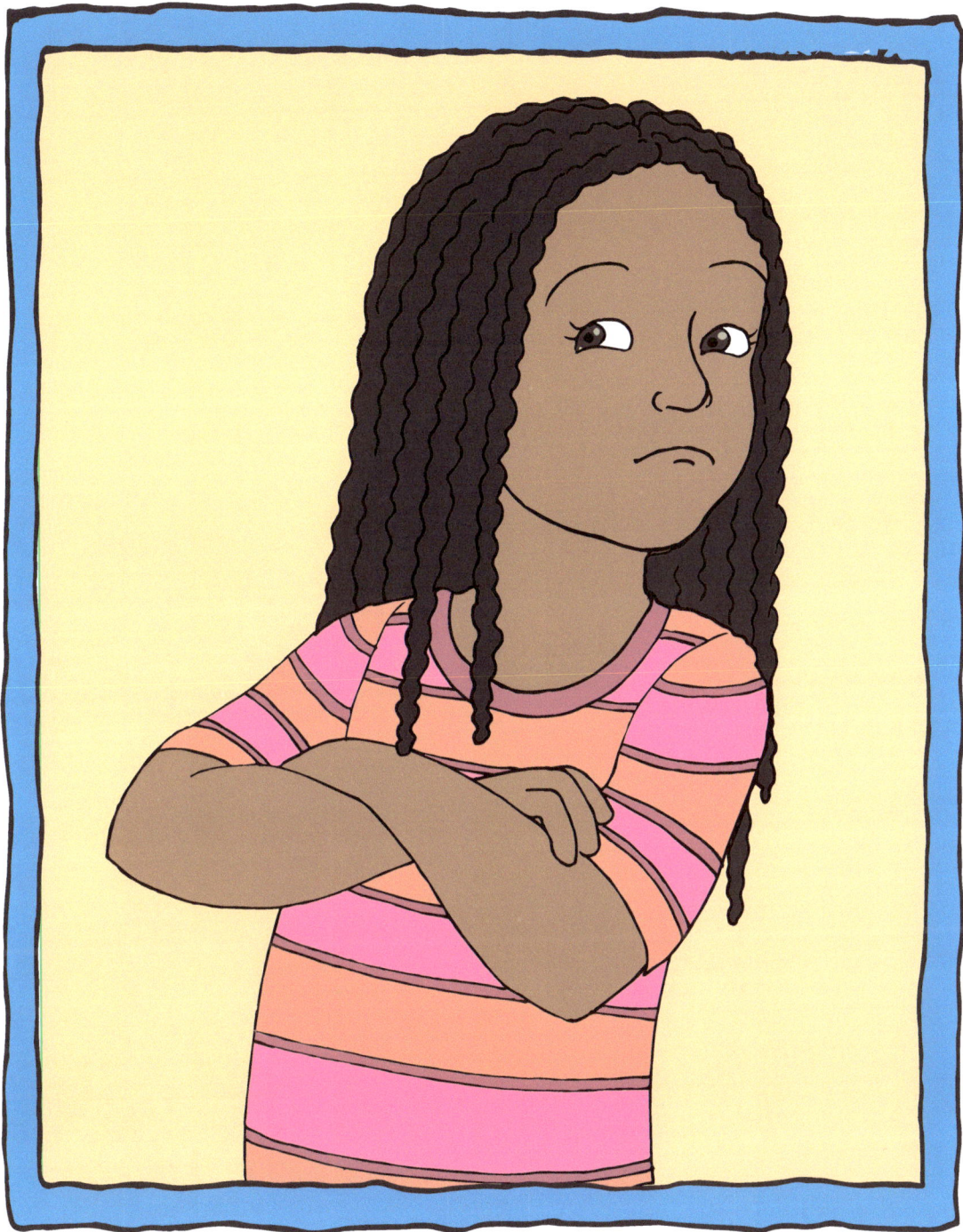

... and some that I don't.

When I eat nutritious food, I have ENERGY, and my brain, blood, bones, and muscles are HEALTHY and STRONG.

But is the food I like to eat healthy?

HEALTHY FOOD can be delicious and make my body feel GREAT!

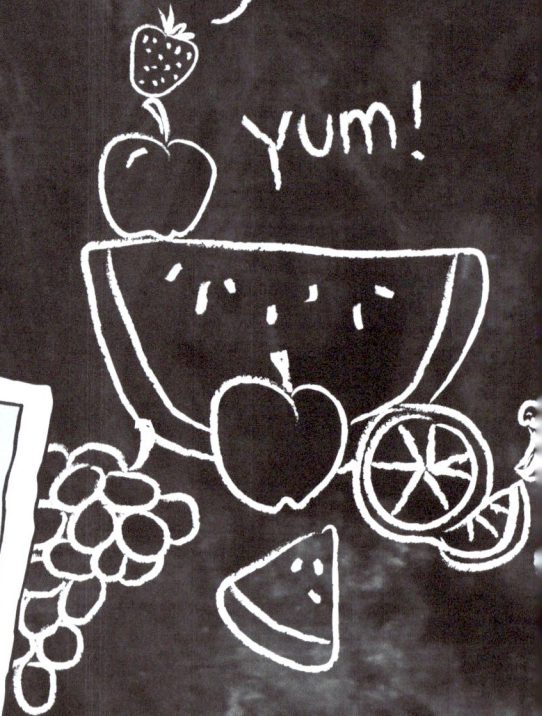

Healthy Food

Yum!

The more sugar we eat, the more we want.
Sugar causes the brain to release a chemical that creates a craving for more and more sugar.
Yikes!
Do you remember feeling sick after eating a lot of sugar at a party or on Halloween?

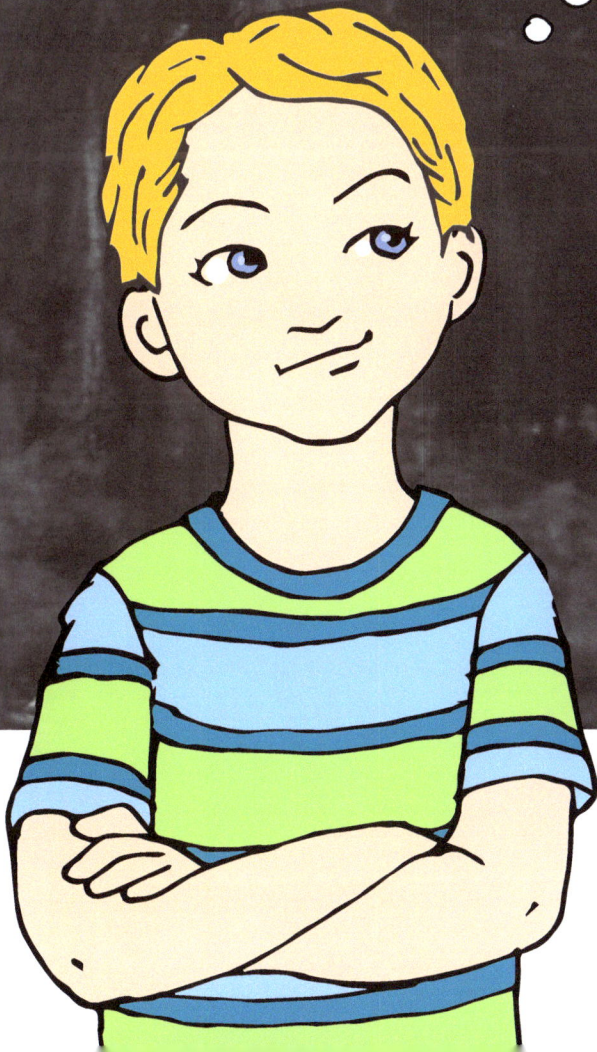

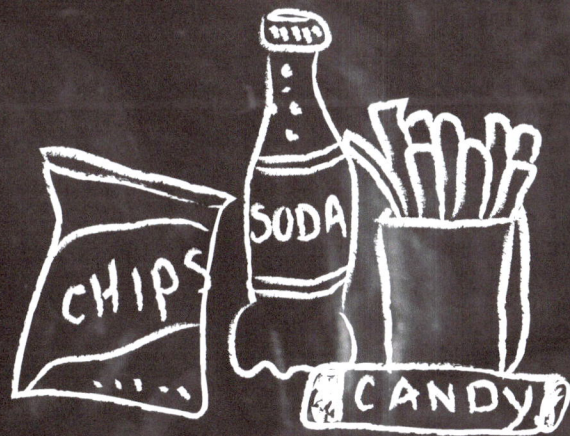

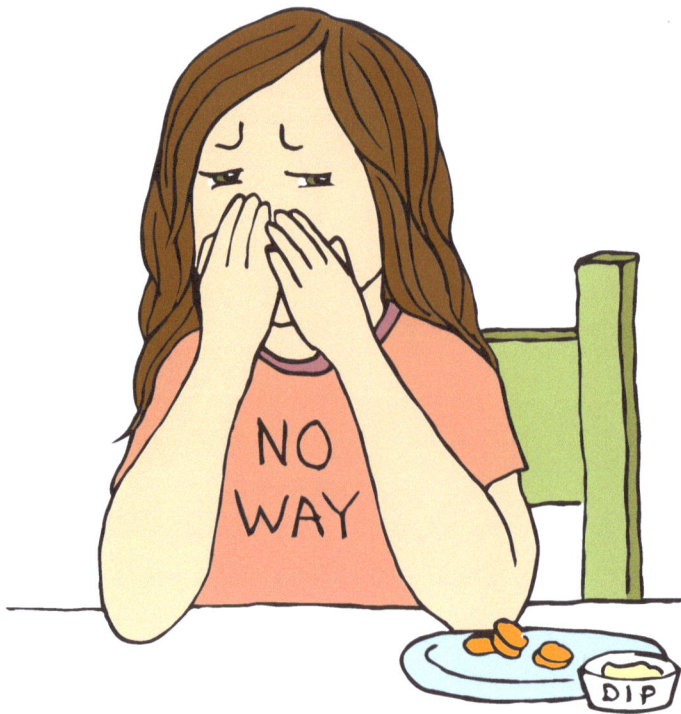

What if I don't like a healthy food?

Wouldn't it be crazy if HEALTHY FOOD that I don't like became food that I do like?

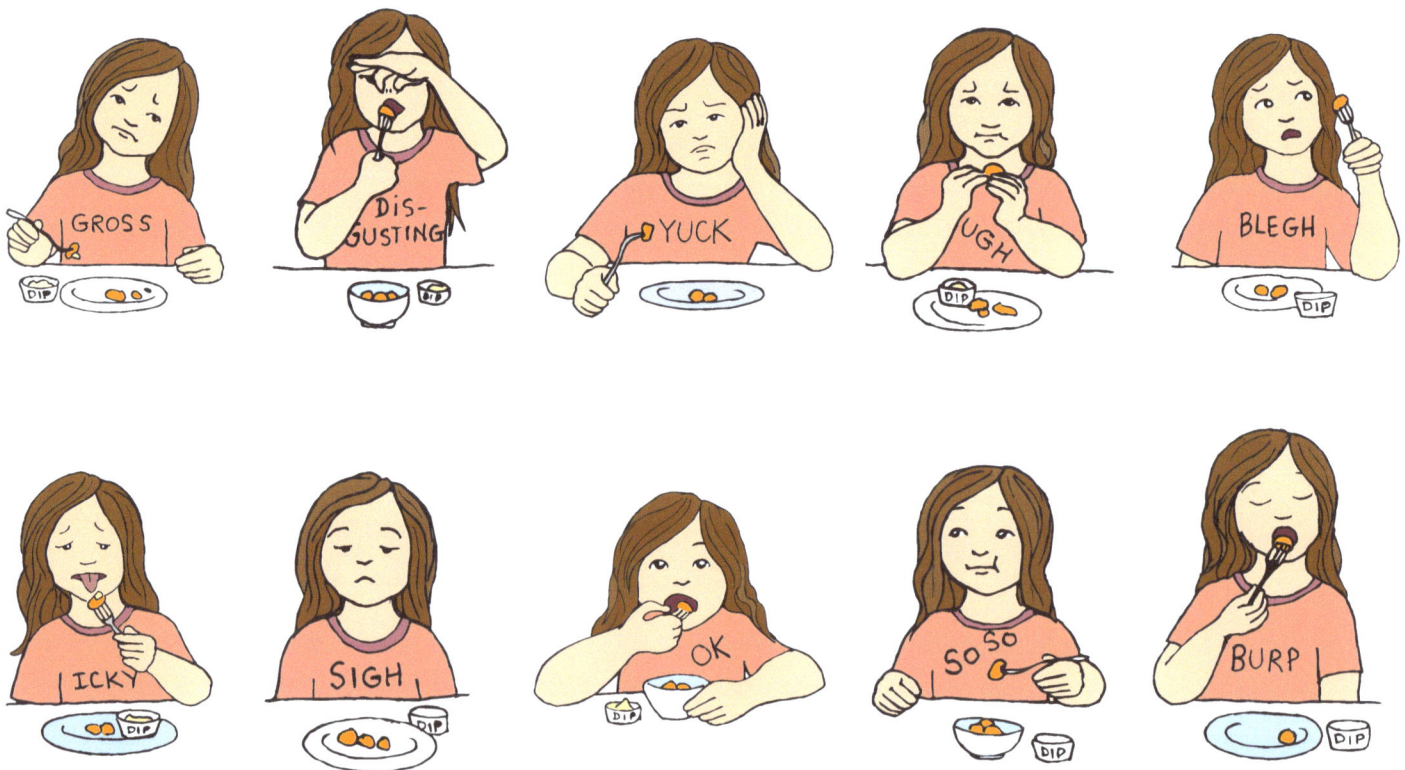

This can happen!

FOOD SCIENTISTS made an amazing discovery:

We can actually CHANGE our tastes

(with a little practice) to become healthy eaters.

It's called an ACQUIRED TASTE.

In an experiment, when kids TRIED a new food that they did not like for at least fourteen days in a row (yes, that means taking a bite), they changed their tastes and began to LIKE that food. But the kids who only tried it once and gave up continued not to like the food. Amazing!

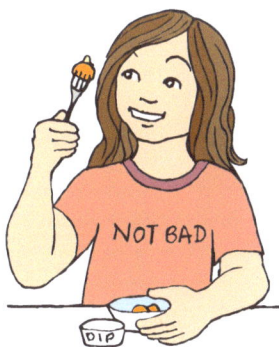

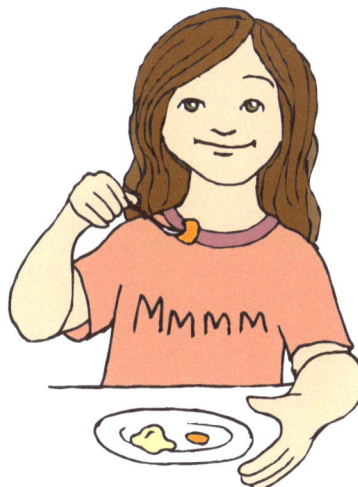

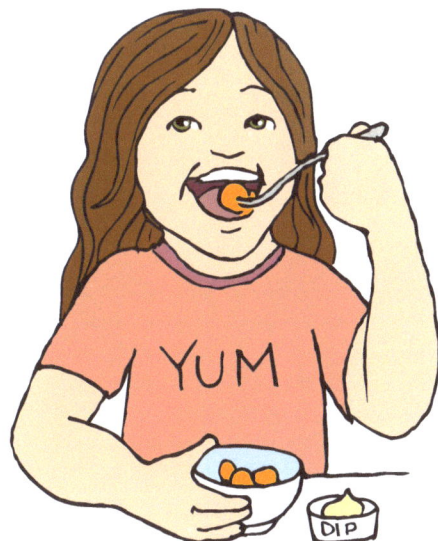

Healthy eaters eat a balanced diet, which means eating a variety of foods in the right AMOUNTS to keep us happy and healthy!

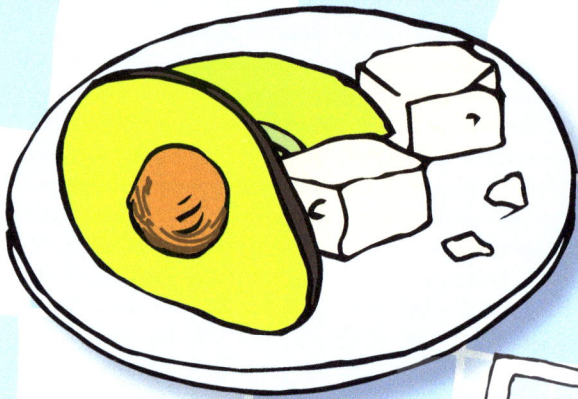

Pick LOW-FAT DAIRY. Yogurt is yummy, but steer clear of high-sugar dairy. Try skim and lowfat milk and cheeses.

Choose HEALTHY FATS such as AVOCADO to supply energy and add flavor. Try plant oils (olive, canola, sunflower), nuts, nut butters, and seeds.

Drink LOTS of WATER. Did you know we lose water every day breathing, crying, sweating, going to the bathroom, and exercising?

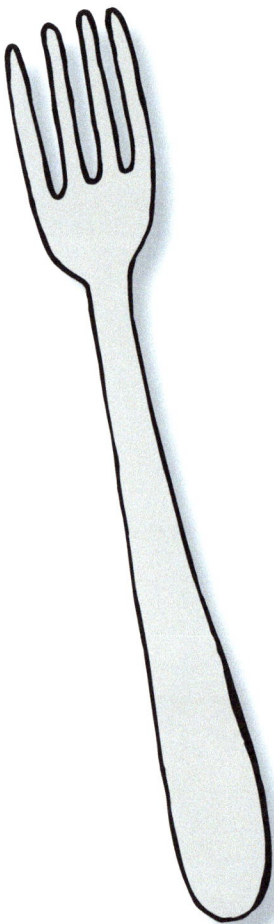

MY BALANCED PLATE

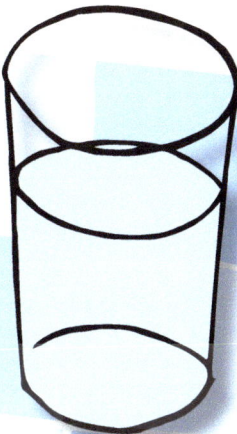

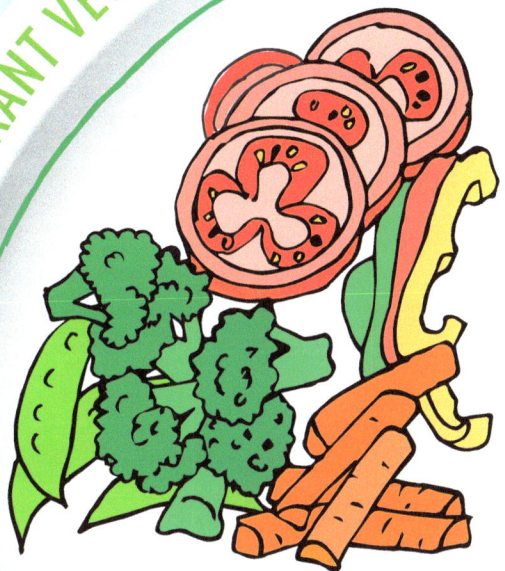

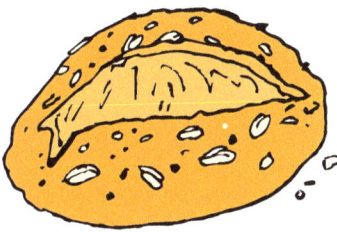

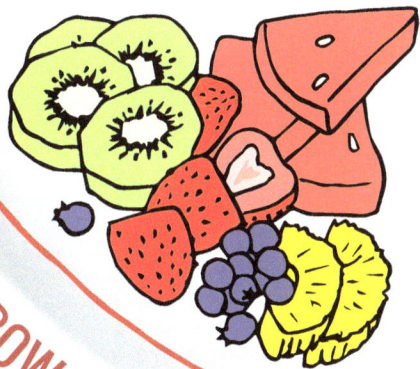

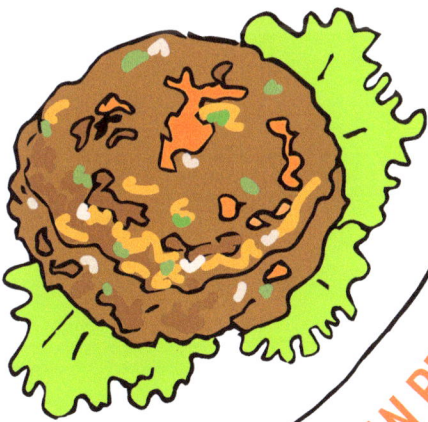

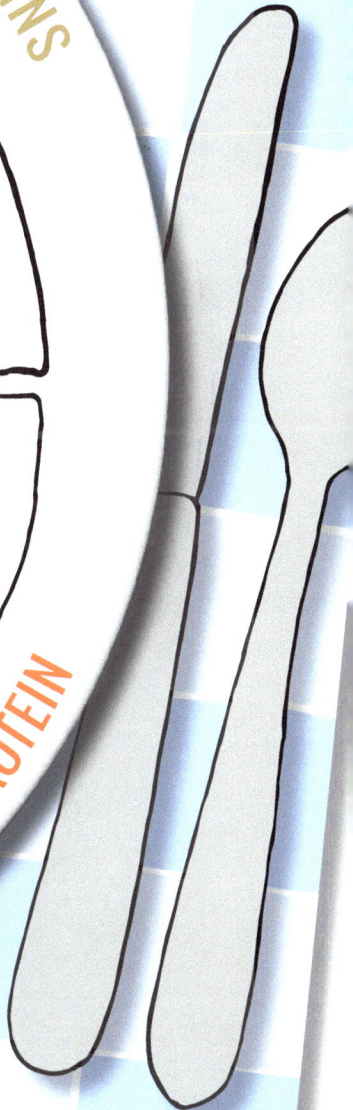

VIBRANT VEGGIES

WHOLE GRAINS

RAINBOW OF FRUIT

LEAN PROTEIN

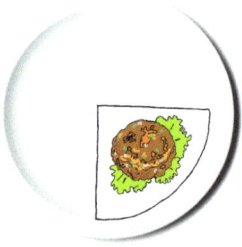

The best way to start the day is with PROTEIN. Protein is important because it keeps us full longer and feeds our muscles and brains. If we eat eggs or a protein smoothie for breakfast, we will feel better all morning, focus at school, and have lots of energy for recess.

Proteins are found in:

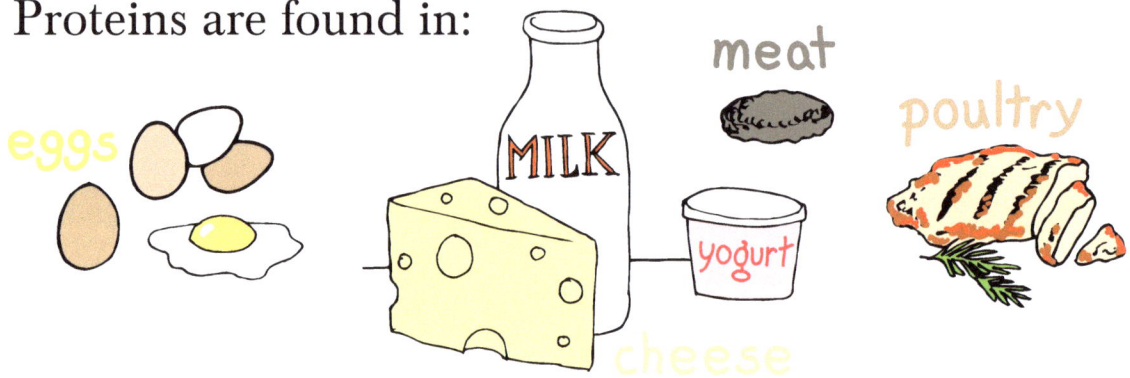

eggs

MILK

meat

poultry

yogurt

cheese

and from plants, such as:

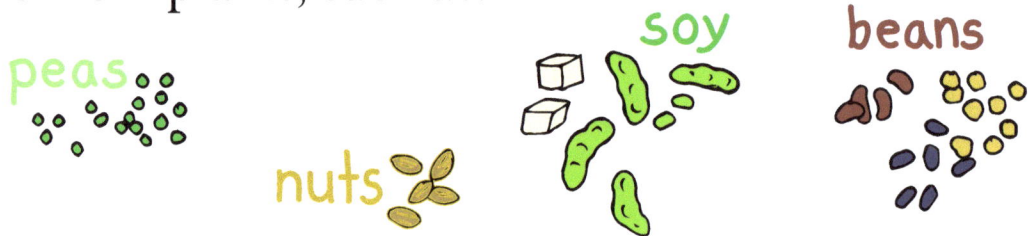

peas

nuts

soy

beans

YAY PROTEIN!

Kids should eat about half of their body weight in grams of protein a day. So if you weigh 60 pounds, you should eat about 30 grams of protein each day.

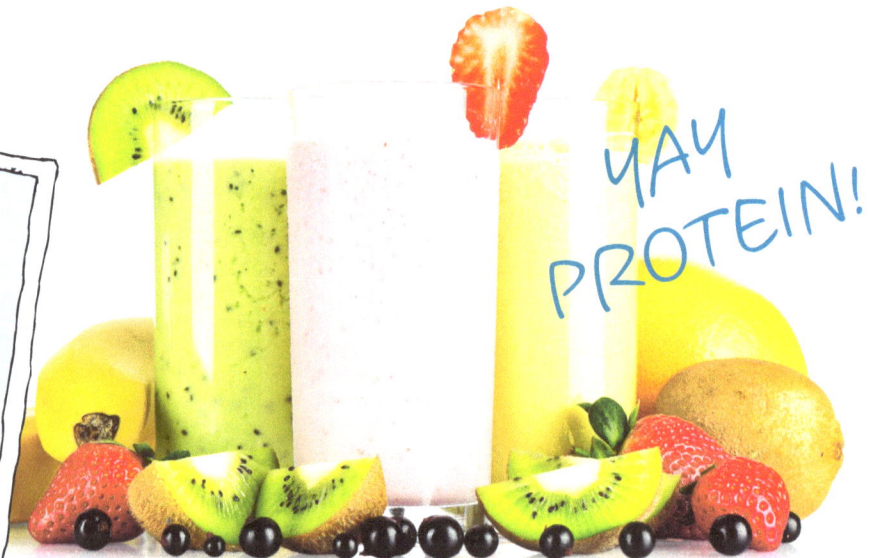

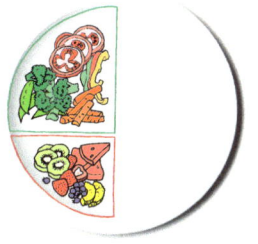

Every day we should eat **LOTS** of delicious

VEGETABLES and **FRUITS**

in a rainbow of colors.

Food scientists have discovered that fruits and vegetables —especially brightly colored— help to prevent illness and keep our bodies and brains healthy and strong. Each color gives us different vitamins and minerals.

Cooking veggies in too much water gets rid of all the good stuff because the vitamins leak into the water. Instead of boiling them, try steaming and roasting vegetables just until tender.

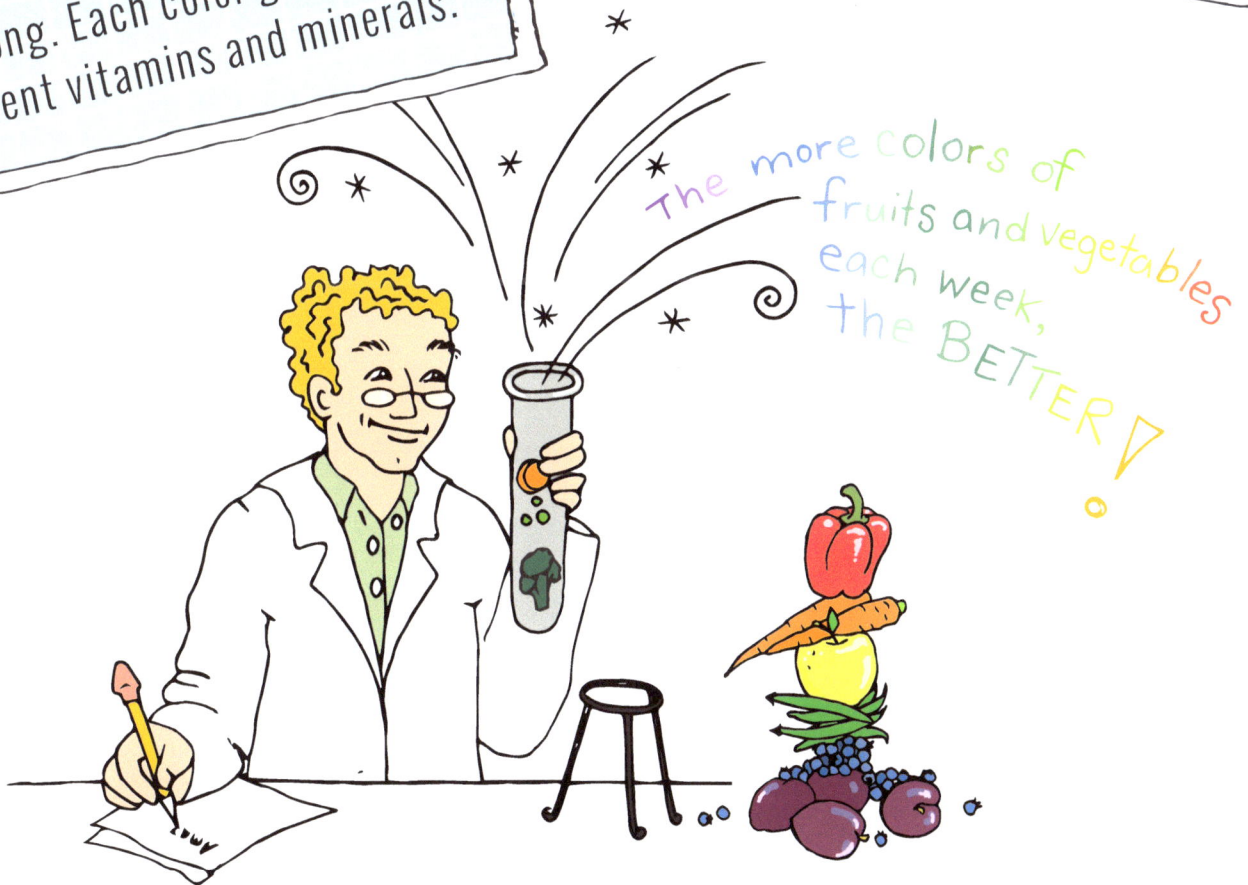

The more colors of fruits and vegetables each week, the BETTER!

Here's a rainbow: red peppers, orange carrots, yellow apples, green beans, blueberries, and purple plums!

One of the best things we can do for our body is:

EAT LESS SUGAR!

When we eat food and drinks with added sugar we
feel tired quickly, crave more sugar,
and feel unsatisfied all day.

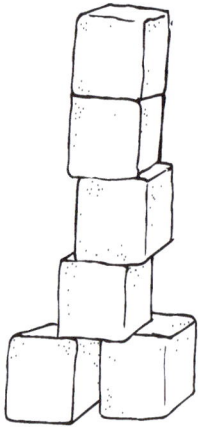

Each day, eat LESS than
6 teaspoons of sugar
(about 25 grams).
1 teaspoon = about 4 grams
of sugar

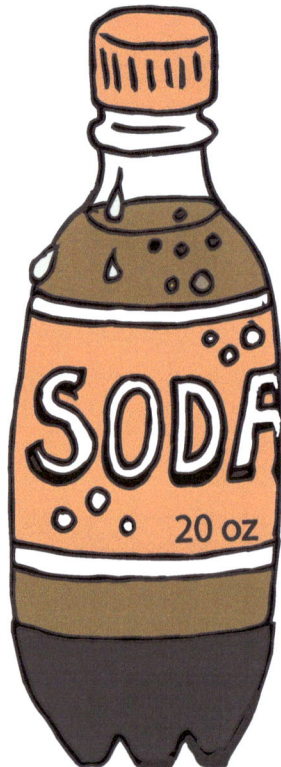

SODA

20 oz

16 TEASPOONS

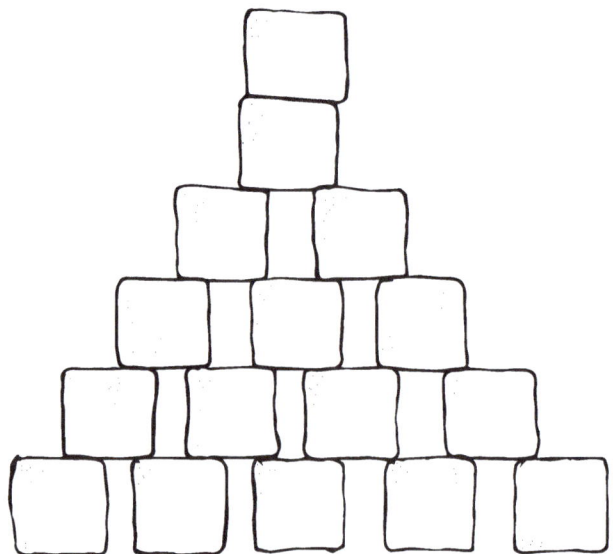

DRINK LOTS OF WATER.

Water gives our bodies a shower from the inside out. Isn't a nice, cold glass of water refreshing?!

Try putting cucumbers, oranges, lemons, or berries in water–*delicious!*

Mmm, WATER with berries.

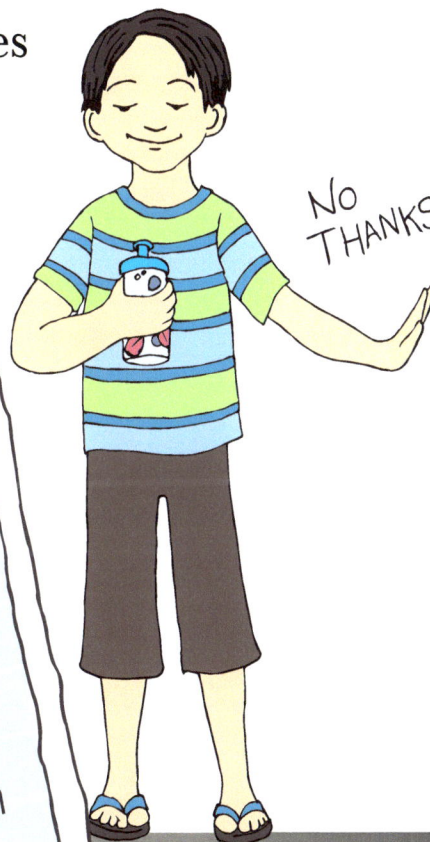

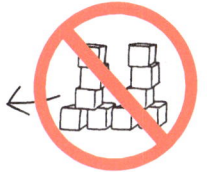

NO THANKS!

SUPER POWER DRINK

AVOID JUICE!
Even 100% fruit juice throws away the healthy fiber and nutrients, the best parts of the fruit, but leaves the SUGAR. It takes 3-4 oranges to make just 1 glass of orange juice. You wouldn't eat 4 oranges for breakfast, would you? Oranges contain FIBER, which prevents sickness, keeps you regular, and fills you up so you're less likely to eat unhealthy food.

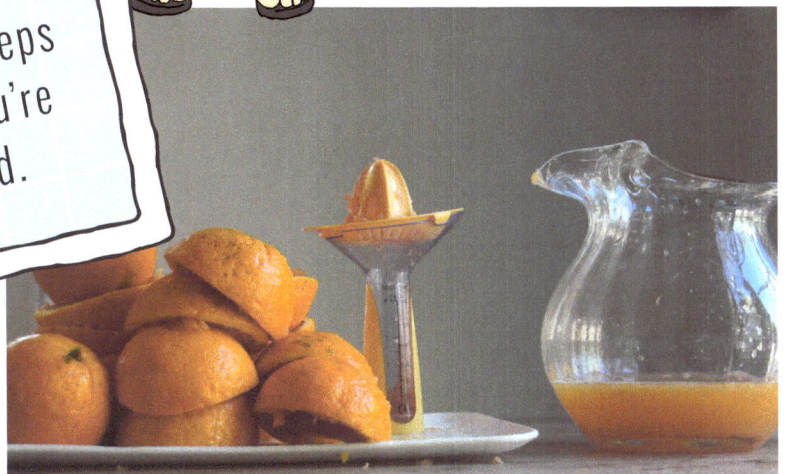

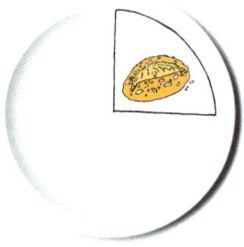

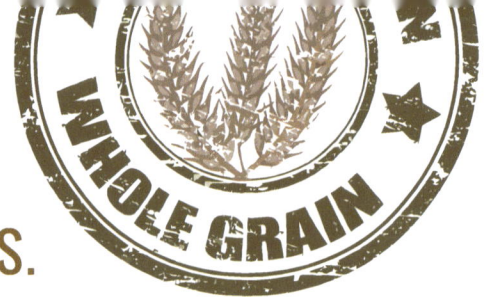

EAT WHOLE GRAINS.

Whole grain bread, whole wheat pasta, and brown rice give us ENERGY and FIBER, which helps to clean out our bodies.

Ask an adult if they know what "WHOLE-GRAIN FOODS" are.

You can explain that these foods use WHOLE seeds from plants, which have all the good stuff–the fiber and the nutrients.

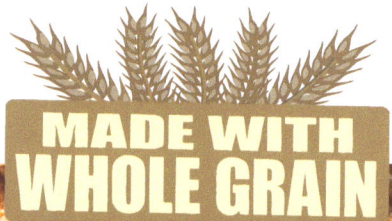

WHOLE GRAIN

MADE WITH WHOLE GRAIN

Look for the words "whole grain" or "whole wheat" on the package. "Wheat flour" is not whole grain, even the word "multi-grain" does not mean it is "whole." Refined grains, such as white bread, regular pasta, and white rice are stripped of important nutrients and fiber and act like sugar in our bodies.

A balanced diet also means eating the right AMOUNT of food and calories and staying active.

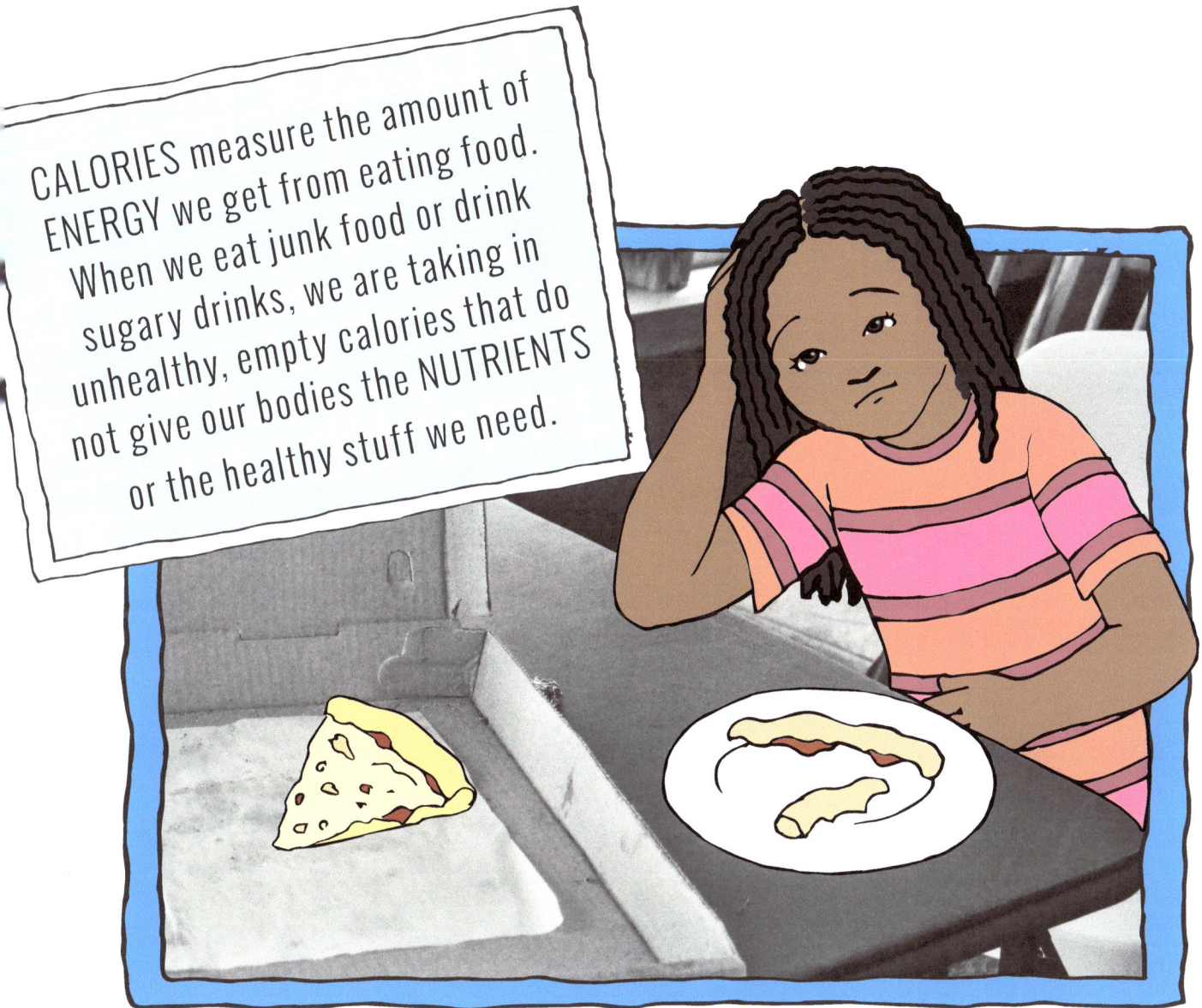

CALORIES measure the amount of ENERGY we get from eating food. When we eat junk food or drink sugary drinks, we are taking in unhealthy, empty calories that do not give our bodies the NUTRIENTS or the healthy stuff we need.

If I ate an entire pizza pie, I wouldn't feel good.

We want to eat only what we need to give us energy,

not a lot more or a lot less.

THAT'S A LOT TO REMEMBER.

Where do I even begin?

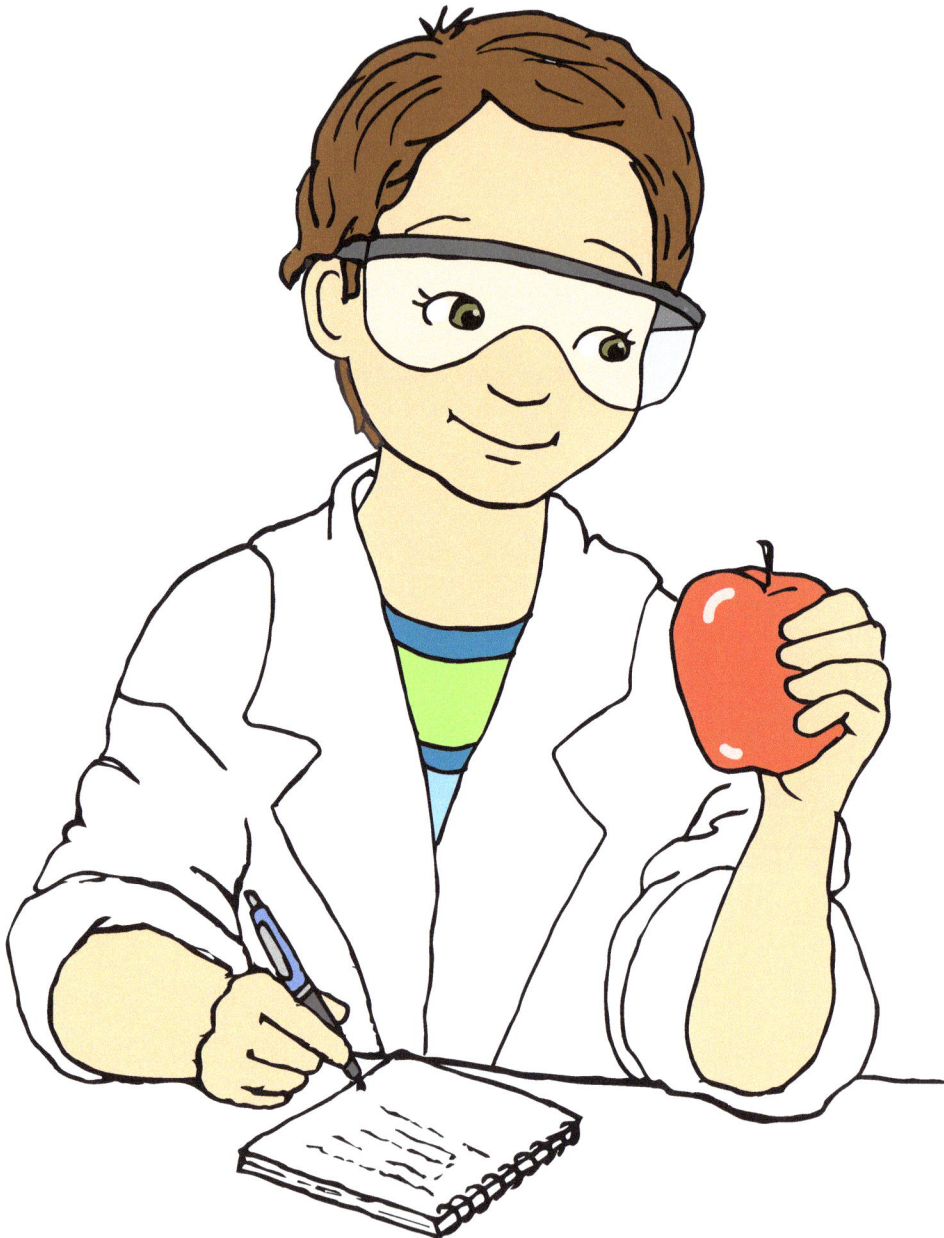

I can be my own food scientist and experiment with different ways to be a HEALTHY EATER.

I can create my very own FOOD JOURNAL and write down: **WHAT I EAT,** **HOW IT TASTES,** **NEW FOODS I TRY,** **MARKETS I VISIT,** and **RECIPES I FIND.**

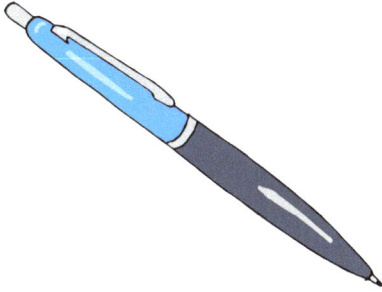

I can help create a **FAMILY RECIPE JOURNAL**

I can be a detective and look for clues in my journal to learn how to eat healthier.

Monday: We baked yummy cupcakes with whole wheat flour and fruit.

Tuesday: Today we tried a new vegetable I had never even heard of before, ARUGULA - it was a little peppery but pretty good.

Wednesday: had a piece of my friend's birthday cake, tomorrow I'll have a frozen fruit popsicle.

Chefs and food scientists have teamed up and shared hundreds of healthy and tasty recipes at pinterest.com/MyPlateRecipes.

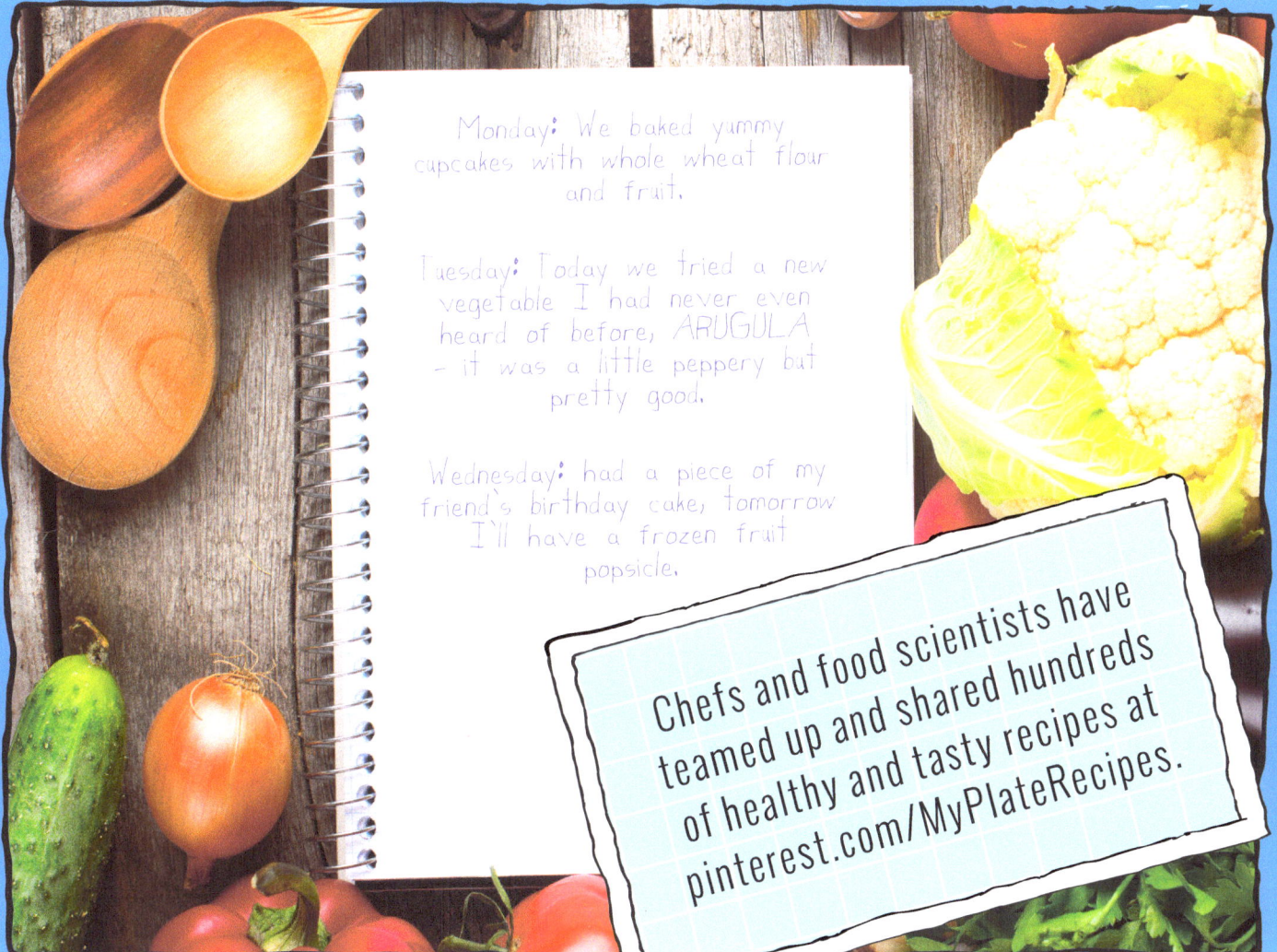

I can try the **TASTE 14 CHALLENGE.** I'll try one healthy food I do not like for 14 days in a row (along with a flavor I do like) to see if I start to like it.

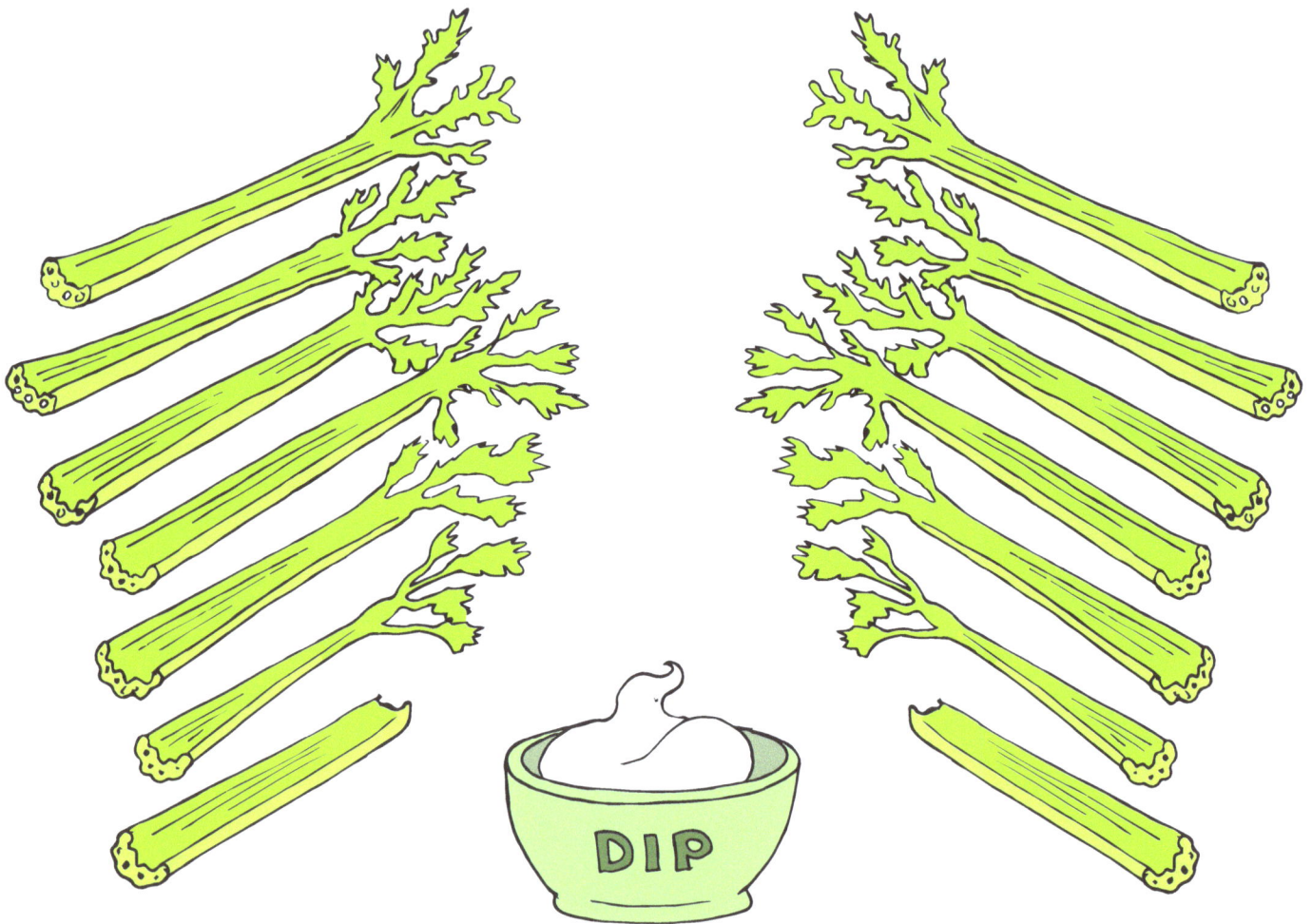

Just a few bites . . .
hey, it's worth it if I start to LIKE it!

I can look at food labels and skip foods with lots of added sugar and long, difficult words such as "high-fructose corn syrup," "artificial colors and flavorings," and "sodium nitrite."

Chances are, if I can't read it,
I shouldn't eat it!

How much sugar is in this food?

Nutrition Facts
8 servings per container
Serving size 2/3 cup (55g)

Amount per 2/3 cup
Calories 230

% DV*

12%	**Total Fat** 8g	
5%	Saturated Fat 1g	
	Trans Fat 0g	
0%	**Cholesterol** 0mg	
7%	**Sodium** 160mg	
12%	**Total Carbs** 37g	
14%	Dietary Fiber 4g	
	Sugars 1g	
	Added Sugar 0g	
	Protein 3g	

10%	**Vitamin D** 2mcg	
20%	**Calcium** 260mg	
45%	**Iron** 8mg	
5%	**Potassium** 235mg	

* Footnote on Daily Values (DV) and calories reference to be inserted here.

The less the better!

Do I know what's in this food?

I can try to eat

more **WHOLE FOOD**, fresh from nature, and

less **PROCESSED FOOD**, which comes in a

package at the store, often with

added sugar and chemicals.

I can plant a garden to have fresh fruits,
vegetables, and herbs to eat.

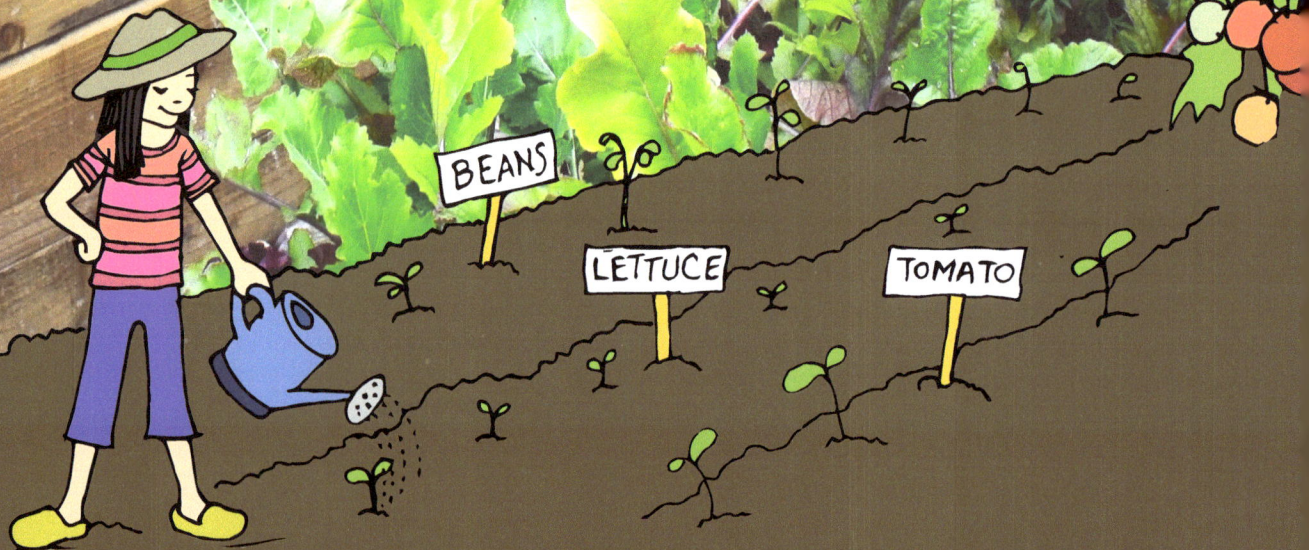

BEANS

LETTUCE

TOMATO

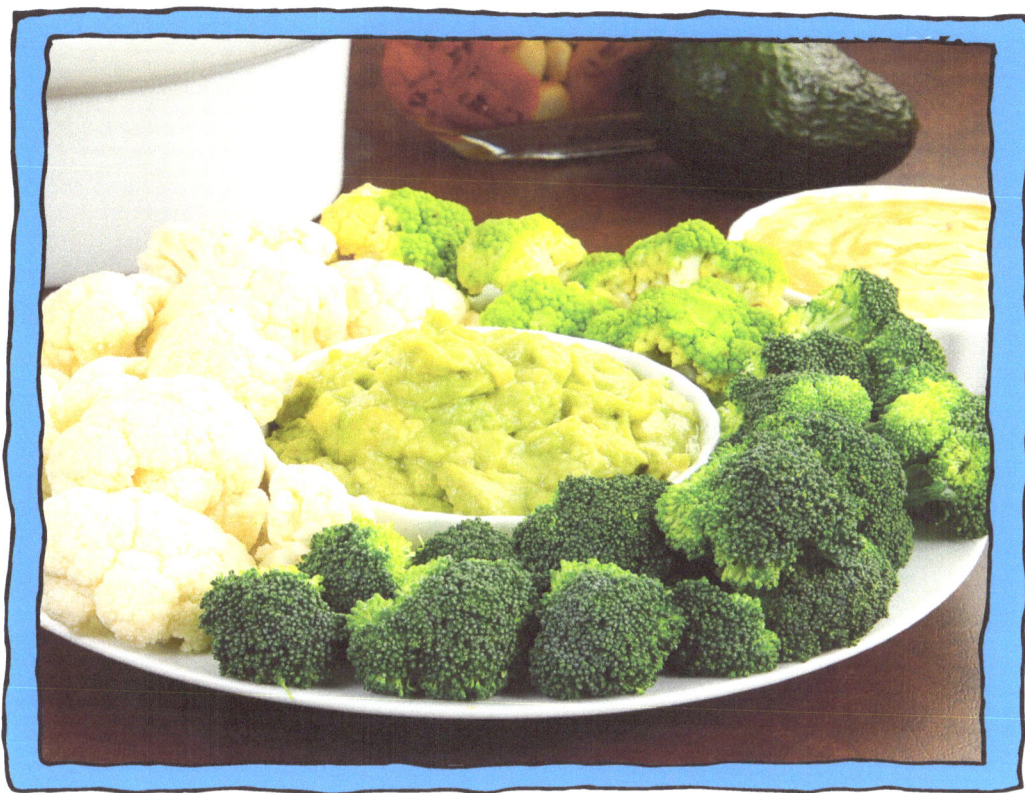

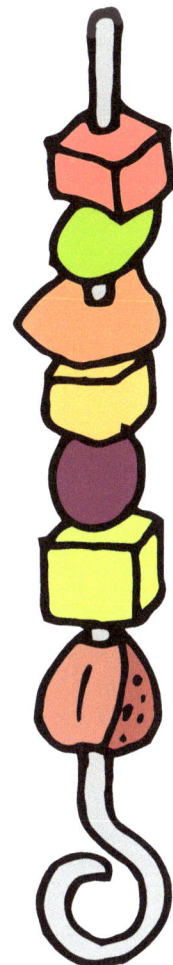

I can be a SMART SNACKER and a
DISCRIMINATING DESSERT EATER. There are so many
scrumptious, healthy choices for snacks:
vegetables with a yummy dip, fresh fruits, and cheese.
For dessert, I can make frozen fruit pops or
bake whole-grain desserts with less sugar.
Hmmmm, I'm getting hungry just
thinking about it.

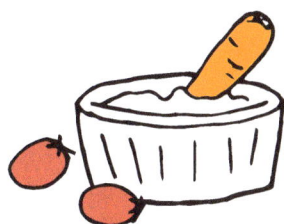

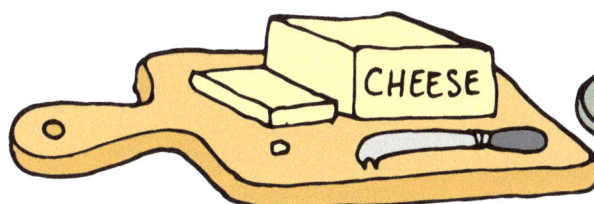

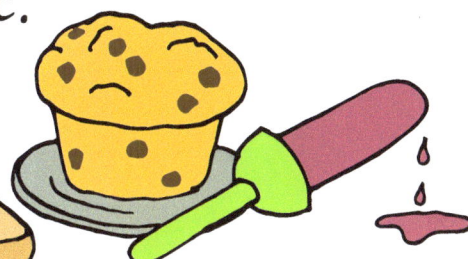

CHEESE

I can make sure that I'm ACTIVE.

WHEN I EXERCISE AND MOVE MY BODY I FEEL GREAT!
EXERCISE KEEPS MY BODY STRONG AND USES UP THE
ENERGY FROM CALORIES THAT I EAT.

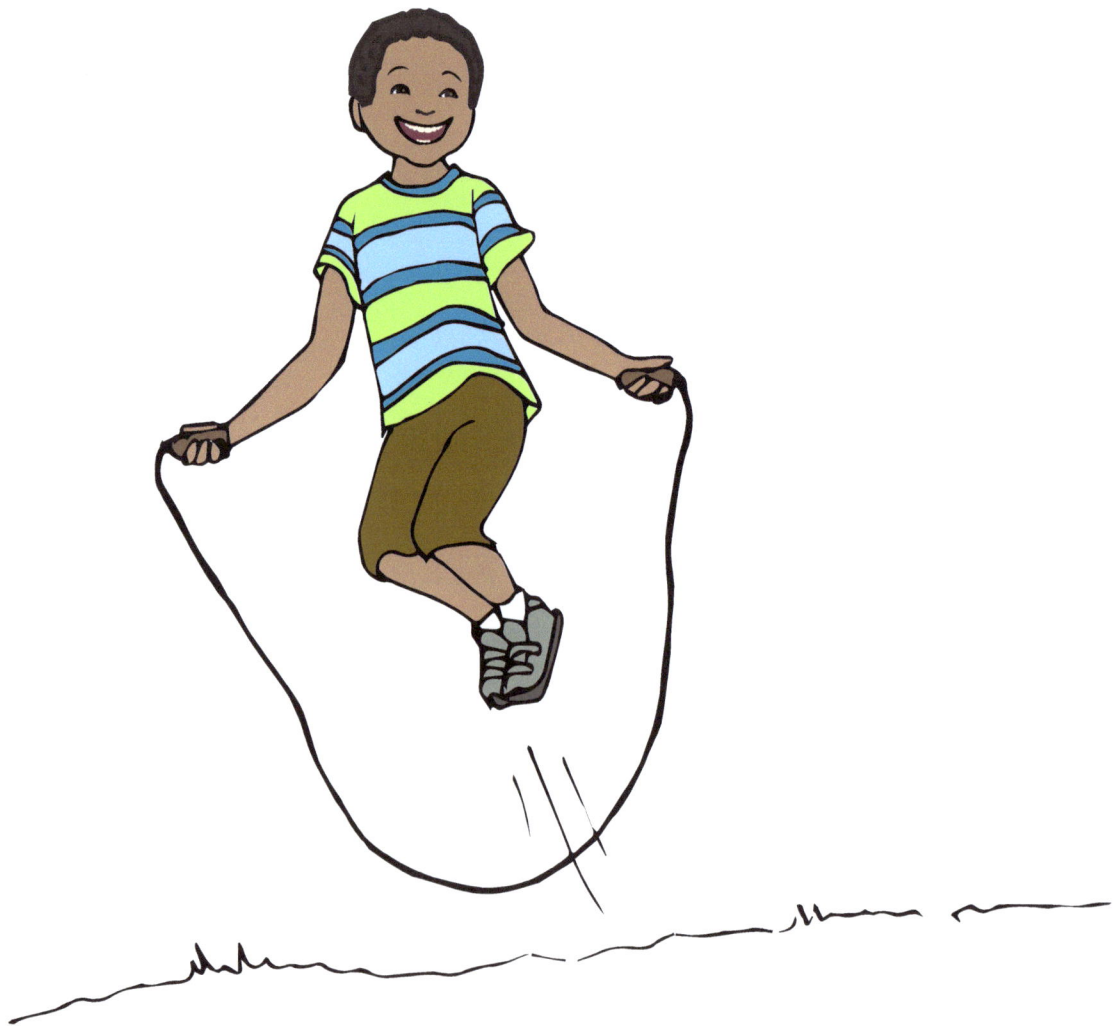

Sample plan:

Put lots of colorful vegetables on my plate.

Start the day with PROTEIN.

Try a healthy food I don't like for 14 days. Keep track in my FOOD JOURNAL.

Jump rope, play outside, be ACTIVE.

Make frozen fruit pops for dessert.

I can start to be a **HEALTHY EATER**

just by making my own plan!

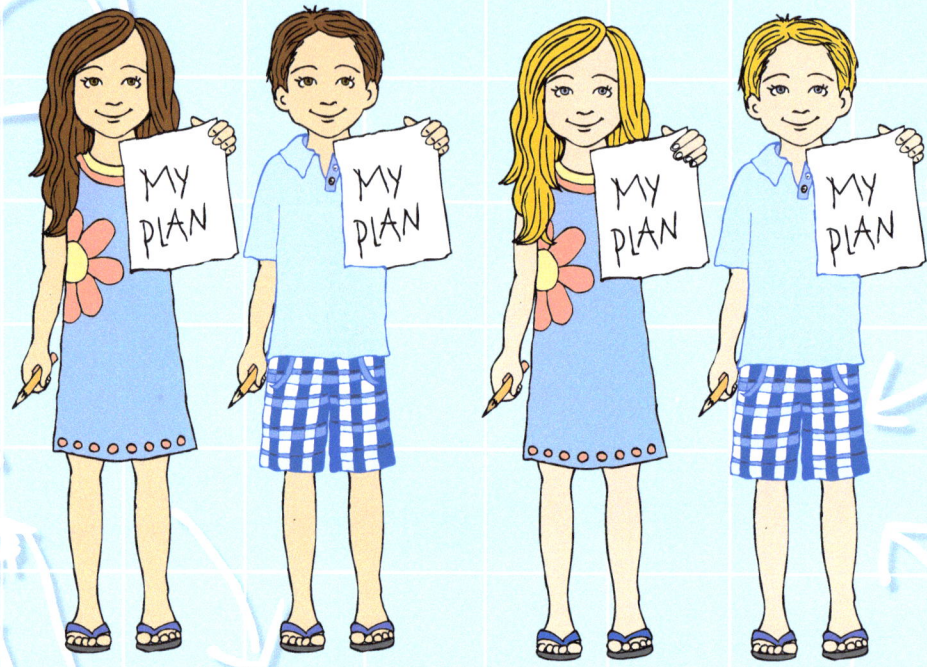

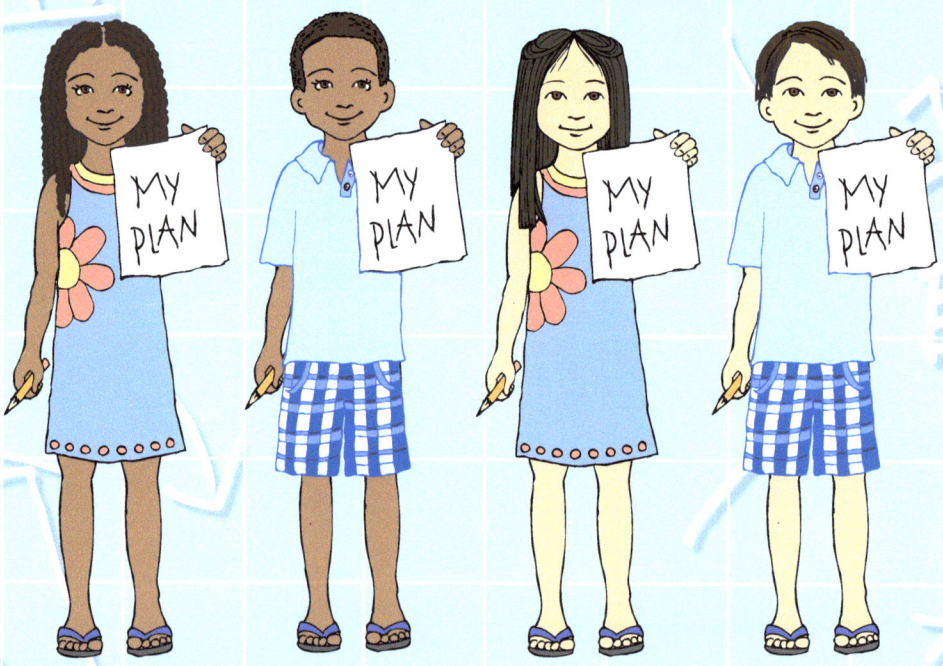

Here is MY PLAN

Other titles in the
HAVE A PLAN Series

WHEN IT'S TIME FOR BED, I HAVE A PLAN

TO CELEBRATE THE HOLIDAYS, I HAVE A PLAN

WHEN I MISS SOMEONE SPECIAL, I HAVE A PLAN

WHEN I MISS MY SPECIAL PET, I HAVE A PLAN

TO BE SAFE AT HOME, I HAVE A PLAN

TO BE SAFE ON THE GO, I HAVE A PLAN

TO KEEP MY BODY SAFE, I HAVE A PLAN

WHEN MY PARENTS DIVORCE, I HAVE A PLAN

WHEN MY PARENTS SEPARATE, I HAVE A PLAN

AND MORE

New titles added regularly at
www.littleBLUEPRINT.com

All titles are available ready-made and personalized

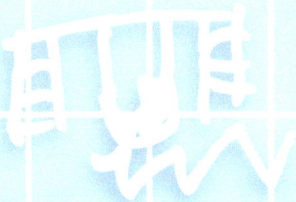
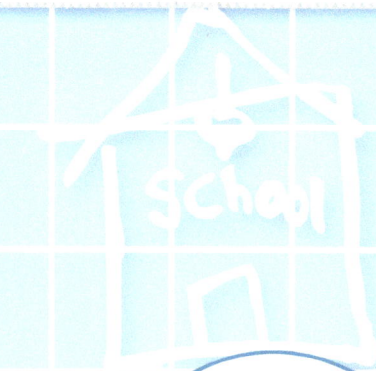
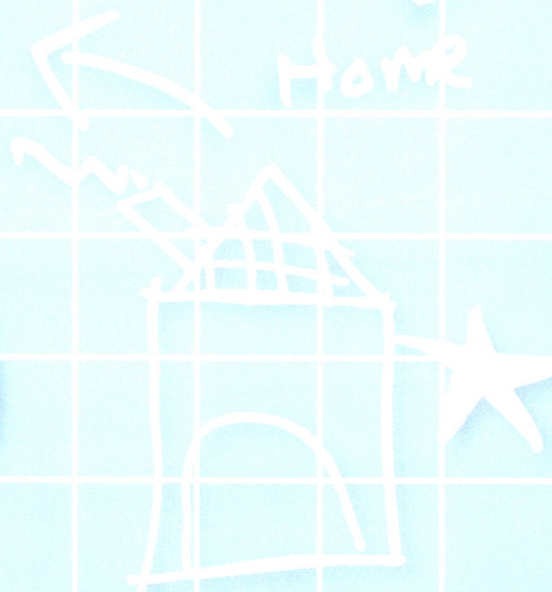
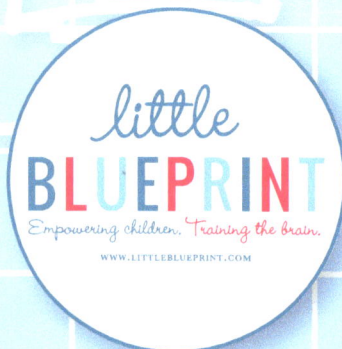

little
BLUEPRINT
Empowering children. Training the brain.
WWW.LITTLEBLUEPRINT.COM

www.ingramcontent.com/pod-product-compliance
Lightning Source LLC
LaVergne TN
LVHW072101070426
835508LV00002B/209